Aphrodite
Bread & Wine Diet

Diet Books by K.J.R Alexander

Love Your Diet Series:

Light Fantastic

Aphrodite Bread & Wine Diet

Calorie Counter
Maximum Calories: The Goldilocks Paradigm

Love Your Diet Recipes

Vitamins & Minerals

The Ancient Foods Diet

Alexander Love Your Diet Series

Aphrodite

Bread & Wine Diet

K.J.R Alexander

Credits

Public domain and free use photos and illustrations provided courtesy of
Wikimedia Commons and the USDA , United States Department of Agriculture.
See listed credits in *Photos & Illustrations* and *Bibliography*.

Factual data is extrapolated and compiled from USDA research and
information publications. See *Bibliography.*

This diet is a sound, balanced, nutritious program. However, no part of this diet
is to be interpreted as replacing professional medical programs, advice, or
prescriptions. Ask your doctor if you have questions.

For a Toast to the Good Times
Of Love, Laughter, Art, Beauty,
Good Food, Bread and Wine for All

Contents

Charts and Tables

1

Aphrodite
Goddess of Love and Beauty

Aphrodite (*A fro dye´ tee* or *A fro dee´ tee*) was the ancient Greek goddess of love and beauty, the power behind love in gods and humans. In Ancient Rome, she was known as Venus. In legend, she was born from the sea and her power of beauty was so great that any man who saw her fell in love with her.

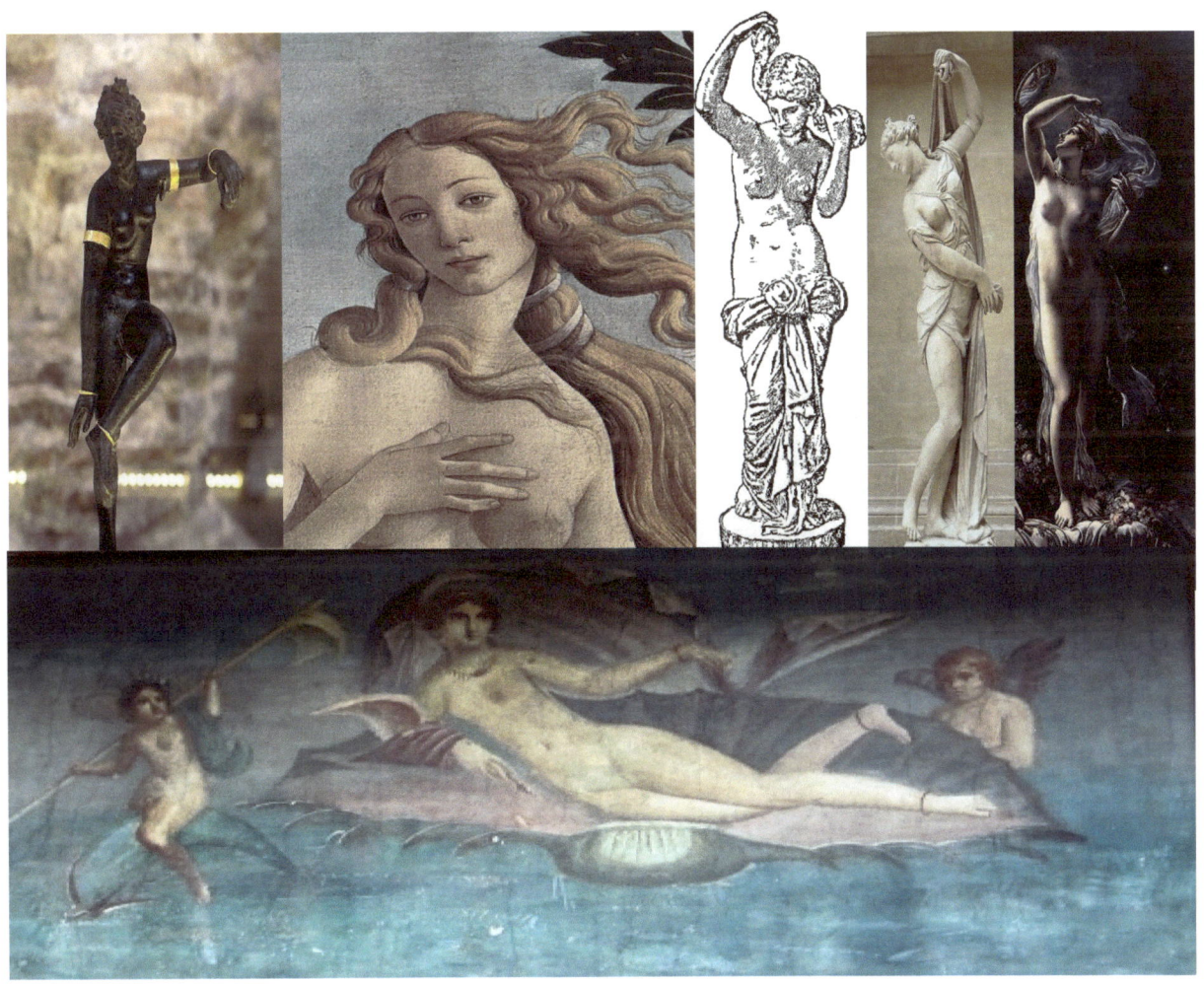

See *Photographs and Illustrations* for photo information.

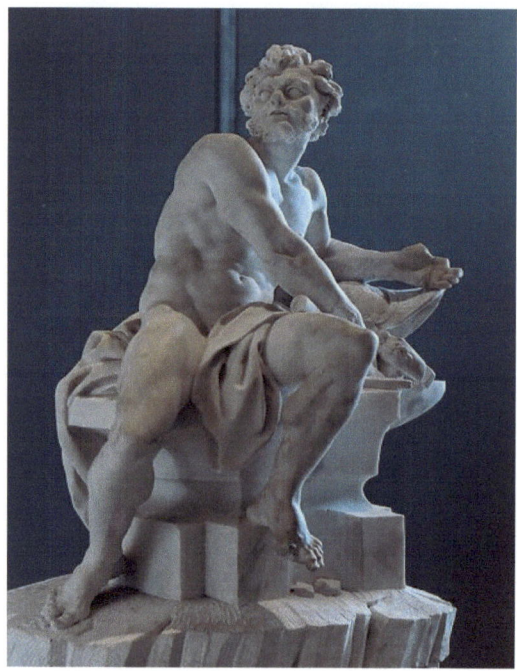

Zeus, the god of gods, feared that Aphrodite's great and powerful beauty would cause fighting among the other gods of Mount Olympus, so he married her to the homely, modest Hephaestus, the god of technology and craftsmen, sculptors and goldsmiths, fires and volcanoes. Hephaestus made beautiful jewelry for Aphrodite, including the magical girdle belt she wore, the source of irresistible sexual attraction.

Hephaestus, god of arts and crafts, technology and smithing. In Rome, his name was Vulcan.
Photo: Jastrow, 2006

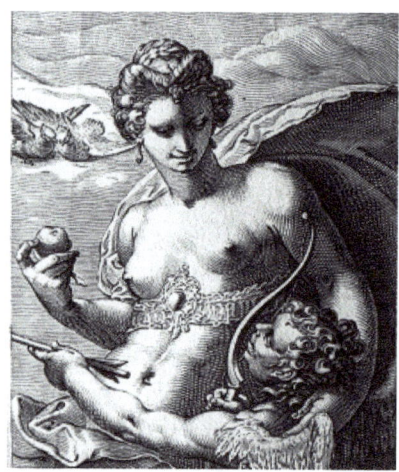

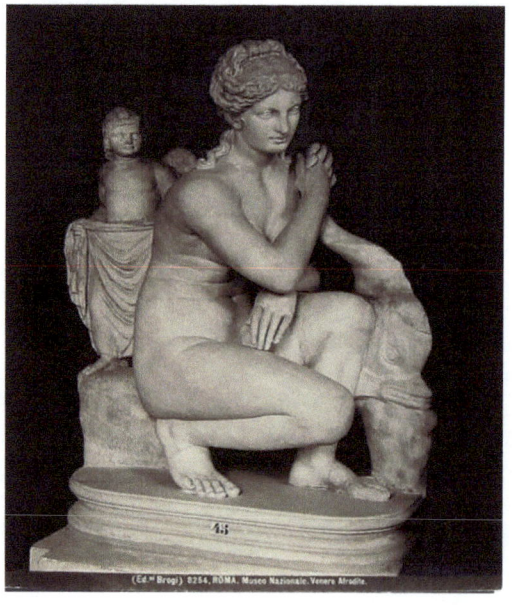

Aphrodite in the girdle by Hephaestus (above) and with son Eros (above and left), god of love and sexual desire. Eros could shoot arrows into gods and humans, causing irresistible love. Engraving above by Jan Saenredam. Statue left by Carlo Brogi.

Goddess Aphrodite was not bound by marriage however, as she pursued love with other gods, such as the strong Ares, god of war, and the young handsome Adonis, god of rebirth and vegetation.

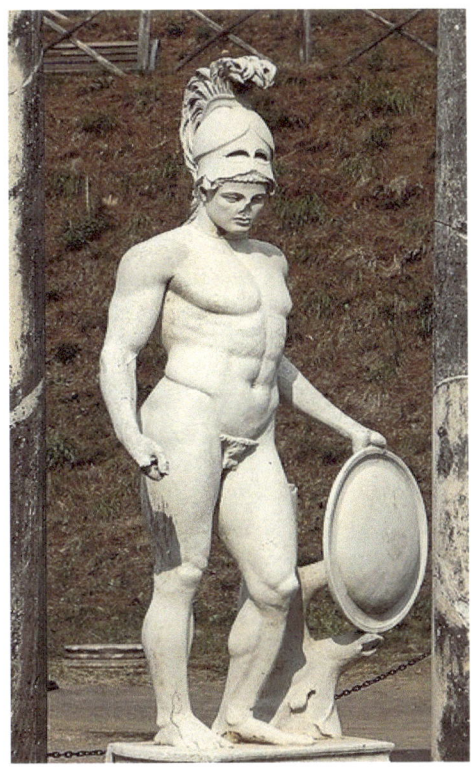

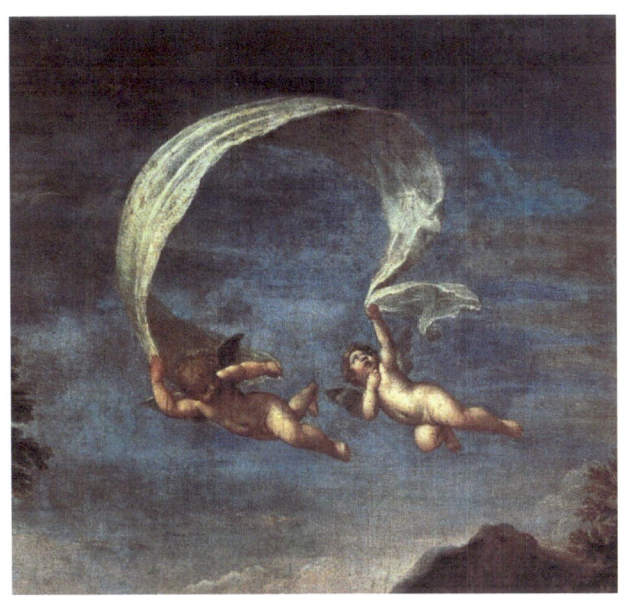

Cupids leading Adonis to Aphrodite.
Painting by Francesco Albani

Ares, god of war.
In Rome, his name was Mars.
Photo: Jastrow, 2006

Adonis, god of rebirth.
Photo: fr. Utilisateur.DS

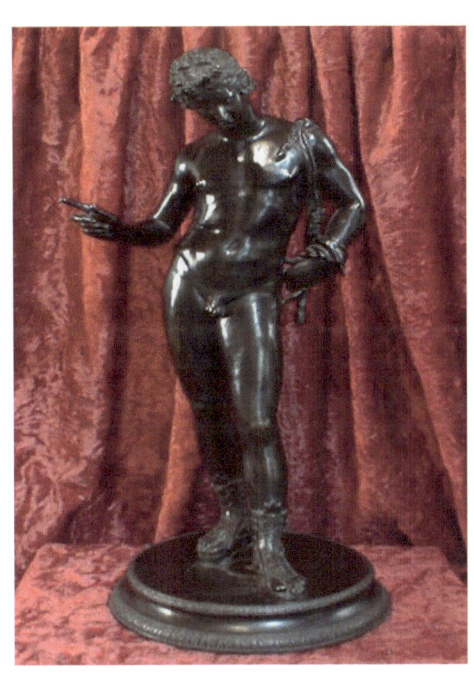

The Death of Adonis.
Sculpture by Giuseppte Mazzuoli
Photo: Mark Thorpe, 1999

Aphrodite discovers the death of Adonis
Painting by Jose de Ribera

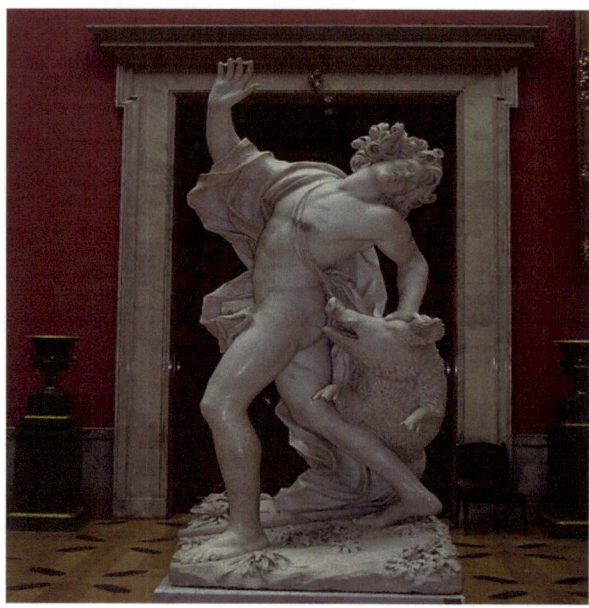

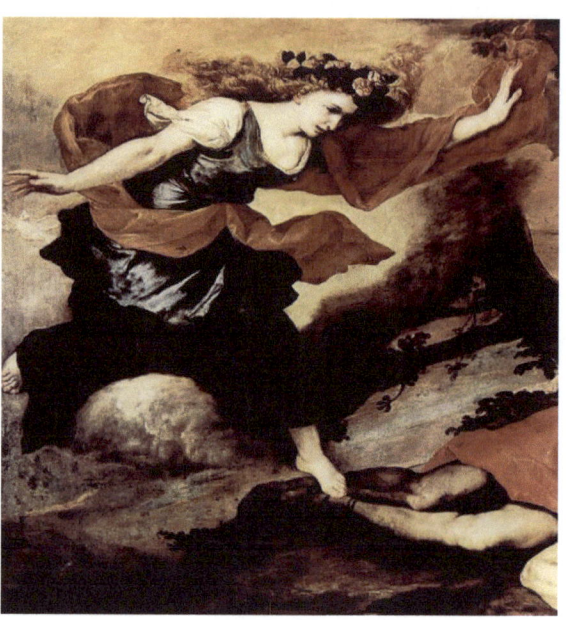

While hunting, Adonis was attacked and killed by a wild boar, perhaps a form taken by a jealous Ares. Adonis then went to the underworld to Persephone, goddess of earth's fertility and queen of the underworld. Aphrodite and Persephone fought over Adonis, each wanting him for herself, until Zeus made them share him equally. Adonis then stayed with Persephone in the world below for six months and Aphrodite in the world above for six months, a process symbolizing the change of seasons and the growth of annual plants.

Adonis lived, died, and lived again in cycles. In ancient times, during the summer Festival of Adonis, he was celebrated by women in Athens who planted rooftop *Gardens of Adonis* with seeds of herbs, wheat, and barley that would quickly grow into plants, then wilt and die in the hot sun. In ceremony, the women would then loudly wail and mourn the death of Adonis, the handsome rebirth and vegetation god.

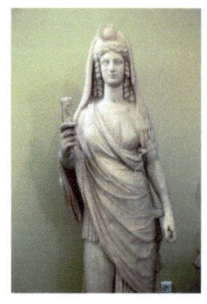

The Awakening of Adonis
by Aphrodite
Painting by John William
Waterhouse

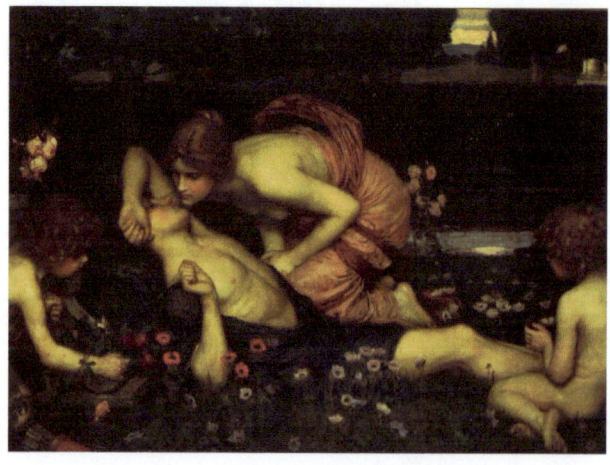

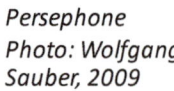

Persephone
Photo: Wolfgang
Sauber, 2009

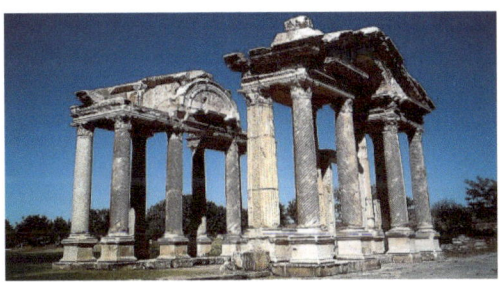

Aphrodisias Tetrapylon
Aphrodite Temple
Photo: M.Chloe Mulderia, 2004

For ancient peoples, myths made life's mysteries comprehensible in characters and stories. In the mythical world of Aphrodite, the purpose and power of love and beauty are symbolized in her relationships:

Aphrodite symbolically gave love and beauty to crafts and arts.
> Her first role, shown in marriage, was to give love and beauty to the crafts, arts, and forging powers of Hephaestus. She was the source for the feelings of beauty in a work of art and was the inspiration behind its creation.

Her positive forces healed the effects of war.
> In her relationship to Ares, the war god, love and beauty tempered and counteracted the destruction of war.

She created renewal and regeneration.
> Her relationship to Adonis sparked winter dormancy to spring renewal. This also symbolized emotional healing and growth after difficulty.

She was the source of attraction, passion, and pleasure for reproduction.
> Eros, one of her children, the god of love and sexual desire, could direct the force of love into humans. In Rome, his name was Cupid. He exists in popular culture today as a cherub who shoots an arrow into the unwary, striking him or her with sudden love at first sight.

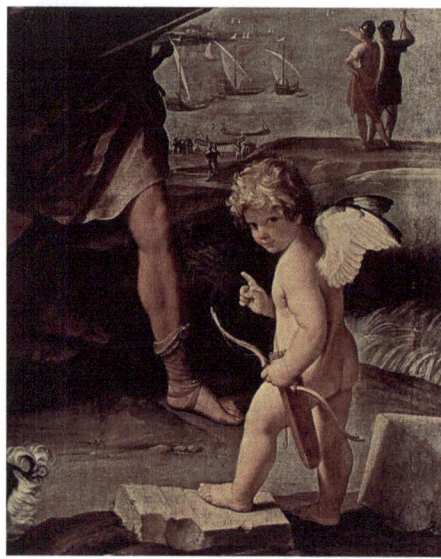

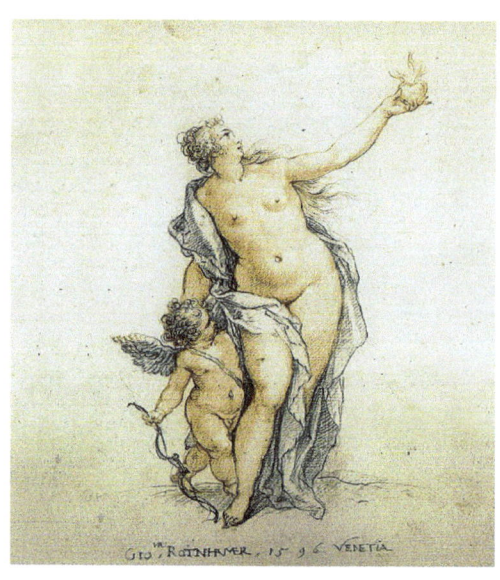

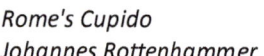
Rome's Cupido
Johannes Rottenhammer

Aphrodite and Eros
Guido Reni

Through the centuries, Aphrodite is seen in many forms as artists and sculptors create her image to portray love and beauty. Not only is she a source of the indefinable something of beauty and its relationship to attraction and love, she fires the passions of life elevated to artistic beauty and harmony.

Any worthwhile pursuit needs the passion and harmony of love and beauty, which give joy and pleasure, make work satisfying, create art, heal sorrows and pain, and continually renew life.

The Aphrodite Bread and Wine Diet is a diet of love and beauty, of positive energies towards harmony and balance. It is a loving and comfortable diet in which you respect yourself and gain confidence. It celebrates the passion of food and the art of dining with pleasure and satisfaction. It will prove that a diet can be enjoyed while losing excess fat. How to do so is revealed in the following pages.

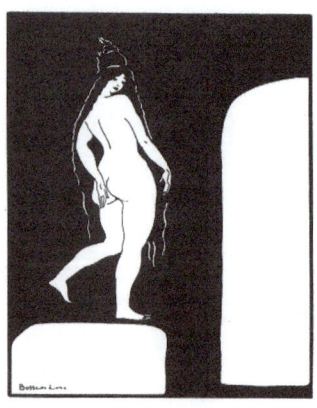

Illustration to Ovid's Art of Love, 1930
Jean de Bosschere, The Love Books of Ovid

2

Code of the Ancient Harvest

The *Aphrodite Bread & Wine Diet* is a revolutionary approach to traditional dieting methods. This diet shows how to eat all kinds of foods, including carbohydrates, while losing that excess fat, without hunger and without necessary exercise. This is accomplished by giving the body the foods it needs for efficient metabolism. These are foods that "tune up" metabolism. (Metabolism is the term for the highly complex processes the body uses to turn food into life energy.)

Looking at all the food in the food environment and then looking at all the overweight people in that environment readily reveals the source of the problem of excess fat and obesity. The basic problem is in the kinds of food everyone is eating. These are foods that stifle metabolic processes, packing on the fat. They dampen down metabolism because they lack the natural nutrients in the proper balance. The body signals for the food it needs with a constant vague or hidden hunger resulting in feelings to eat more. The more this food is eaten, the more the desire to eat, creating a cycle of food addiction.

So what are these foods and what kinds of foods are needed instead? Most would say that the fat causing foods are junk foods, fast foods, high carbohydrate foods, or high fat and sugar foods, and that the good foods would include more fruits and vegetables.

Why aren't people eating more of the healthy food? The answer is that they are *addicted* to fast convenient foods. In addition, many are confused and unconvinced as to *exactly why* the foods are not good. Advertising also promotes foods that produce profit for the corporate food culture. Additionally, most people basically trust the foods they eat. And finally, people are losing the ability to plan nutritious meals on their own. One cannot live on just fruits and vegetables. The predictable outcomes to all of these factors are weight gain and the consequent dilemmas of dieting methods involving punishment and torture. The only options seem to be to gain weight or diet. After dieting, the weight usually comes back, setting up the cycle all over again, while frustrated dieters announce that "diets just don't work."

Something more is needed. That something more is a larger understanding of foods with a new approach to dieting that respects the body without casting sins of greed and laziness, undermining self confidence. By blaming the overweight victims, attention is diverted from the real causes.

Most would agree that natural foods, *real* foods, are needed by the body. But then the understanding breaks down as to what a natural food is. This is because most food is packaged and prepared while anything else is just too complicated. People just know that they need to eat and they're going to eat from what's available. However, there are choices and very pleasant ones. Foods can be chosen that are natural to metabolism.

The body needs certain nutrients, like vitamins and minerals, carbohydrates, proteins and fats. These needs are based in foods eaten since ancient times over thousands of years. These are foods from the times of the Agricultural Revolution as well as the Stone Age. Scientists often explain that foods of the Stone Age, during hunting and gathering, are most compatible to the body. They also say that the grains and other products of the Agricultural Revolution which were cultivated as opposed to growing wild are fattening. This thinking finds its way into many diets. But this is where this diet is significantly different. This diet takes the stance that the body is also adapted metabolically to the many thousands of years of agriculture, to the rich grains and bread, to the cultured fruits and vegetables, nuts, seeds, herbs, spices, milk and dairy, eggs, honey, meats and poultry, along with ale and wine. All these foods are also natural to genetic heritage.

For a model of the foods metabolically compatible, useful is a look at ancient times to the areas around the Mediterranean, to the great agricultural civilizations such as Egypt, Greece, and Rome, progenitors to Western Civilization. (Agricultural civilizations were also developing in Asia and the Americas.) In these sunny warm climates, near waterways, crops of fruits, vegetables, and grains were easily grown. That the body still needs the nutrients in these foods is shown, for example, in the need for Vitamin C in citrus and other fruits, grown in warm climates. Cells are programmed to need all of these foods, to metabolize these foods from ancient times. Cells have the "code" to metabolize these foods. This is the *Code of the Ancient Harvest.*

So what foods or ingredients are not part of this metabolic code? As the kinds of foods available are directly related to the technology of the time, foods change with technology. The technology to culture and grow seeds created the Agricultural Revolution out of the Stone Age. With the Industrial Revolution, machine technology took over agriculture as the primary supplier of food. During this manufacturing process, food content was changed.

A chart showing the time spans involved readily shows that the body, adapted to nutrients since ancient times, is not adapted to the foods manufactured and processed today. The time of the Industrial Revolution is very recent, placed around 1760, with the mechanized spinning wheel in England. The choice of 52,000 (50,000 years plus 2,000) years is based on the general scientific agreement that the human body has not changed much from ancestors 40,000 to 50,000 years ago.

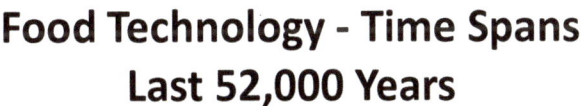

Food Technology - Time Spans
Last 52,000 Years

■ Stone Age: Paleolithic, Old Stone Age 50,000 BC - 12,000 BC

■ Agricultural Revolution & Agricultural Age 12,000 BC - 1760 AD

■ Industrial Revolution & Industrial Age: 1760 AD - 1900 AD

■ Electro-Chemical & Nuclear-Digital Age: 1900 AD - Present

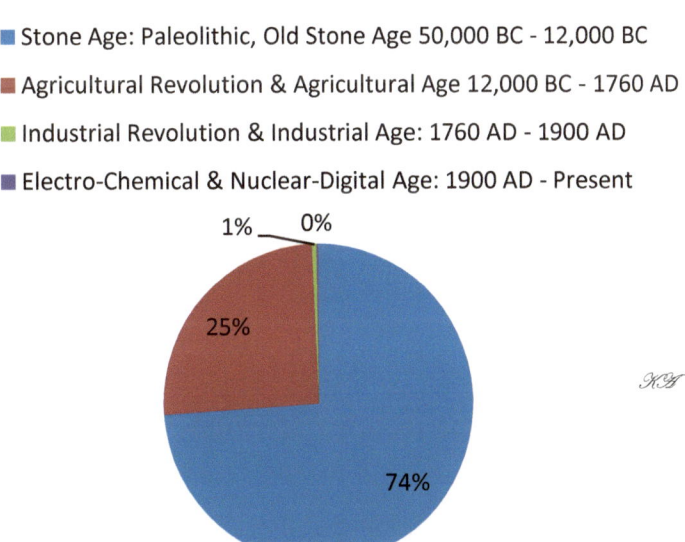

Readily apparent is that manufactured and highly processed foods are very new to the body, developed mostly in the last century with many ingredients seemingly as recent as yesterday. In comparison, this amount of time, the purple area at 0%, is too small to appear on the chart and the Industrial Revolution appears as only a 1% sliver of green.

If one reads the labels and added ingredients on processed foods, regarded along with the epidemic of obesity, it is apparent that foods that are highly processed and changed by manufacturing create a metabolic challenge to the body resulting in excess fat. Therefore, this diet emphasizes foods that are as unchanged as possible by manufacturing. In addition, balance and variety of foods assure nutrition. The reliance on foods from ancient times must be considered to be *cumulative* through the ages. This means that even though people migrated to live in northern climates, with shorter growing seasons and fewer choices, they still need the foods from the warmer climates such as abundant fruits and vegetables. In the *Food History* tables at the end of the chapter, sample lists of these foods show the immense variety of foods to which the body has adapted metabolically and are therefore not inherently fattening. Happily, this expands dieting food choices to include a world of foods.

The ancient civilizations used here are meant only as indicators to the purpose. History changes with new discoveries as times and events are hidden in the ages. However, it is known that peoples traded and shared goods, foods, and technologies across cultures for many thousands of years.

In looking at food history, trends indicate the foods that are metabolically superior for dieting purposes. For example, ancient peoples had to live near waterways for the water and food sources. Consequently, waterbirds, fish, and shellfish were major foods. For this reason, fish, seafood, and poultry, as more ancient, are somewhat more effective diet foods than beef. Other compatible foods are all the varieties of foods developed and cultivated from wild seeds, root foods, berries, and fruit. This includes herbs and spices and all kinds of leafy and pod vegetables. All these natural foods are part of the diet plan and for continued eating after the diet as nonfattening foods. This includes, as all natural foods, beans, rice, potatoes, and sweets such as honey and raw sugar, and rich dried fruits, such as figs and dates.

Food history also indicates the kinds of grain and bread products that are not fattening. This includes whole grains and unleavened (without rising ingredient) and yeast leavened bread. The first breads were unleavened flat breads like tacos, tortillas, and pita bread. (However, the ingredients must be all natural and without saturated fat and baking soda, baking powder, and preservatives.) The Egyptians developed the first ovens for baking yeast leavened breads from wild yeasts by 3,000 BC and made over 40 different kinds of breads and pastries. Yeast is a natural living food and has been used for many thousands of years for making alcoholic beverages and bread. Therefore, yeast leavened foods, bakery fresh, and without preservatives, is compatible and nonfattening. A list for nonfattening grains and bread, developed according to the history of foods, in the order of not fattening to most fattening is also included at the end of the chapter.

Note that since the Agricultural Revolution takes up approximately one fourth of the Food Technology Chart, it can be interpreted to mean that grains and natural bread products at least a fourth of the time, while dieting, will not cause weight gain. This proportion increases after weight loss. It must be emphasized however, that the bread needs to be without chemicals and preservatives, saturated fats, and other manufactured ingredients. It must be bakery fresh without preservatives, and, if white, at least enriched. A good example is french bread from the bakery, fresh that day.

Wine and ale are very much a part of the ancient metabolic heritage. Note in the food tables that all of the ancient civilizations produced wine and ale. The ancient Egyptians produced red and white wines from a half dozen different grapes. Wine bottles were labeled by location, vineyard, and date. Wines were also rated for taste such as good to three times good, sweet and so on. The year 1,344 BC was rated a great vintage year. Egyptian beer or ale was brewed daily from barley and bread grains since before 3,000 BC. (Billard, Editor. *Ancient Egypt. Discovering its Splendors*, listed in *Bibliography*.) Whether modern beers are good diet complements is a matter for personal experimentation, as ale was the primary beverage in ancient times. Again, the more natural the beer or ale, the better. Beverages naturally fermented to alcohol are very much a part of the food heritage from ancestors, from people of the ages, who gained life's reward and comfort from the pleasant euphoria.

Wine in ancient Greece and Rome was part of breakfast along with bread and olive oil. In Rome, the wine was very strong, so was usually diluted with water to prevent wipeout intoxication (not a good way to start, or end, the day). The ancient trio of bread, wine and olive oil are very much a part of our metabolic heritage and therefore essentially nonfattening. Note also, that olive oil, a monounsaturated fat, rather than a polyunsaturated one, is considered to be a good choice today. This undoubtedly traces back, again, to its use in ancient times.

Scan the following tables for an idea of the kinds of foods that feed metabolism and are nonfattening. Helpful lists of foods to eat and not to eat are included with the menus later. The first step in the diet plan however is to stop addiction to the foods that are causing overeating and weight gain. Because most of this food is filled with starchy fillers and sugars, it is referred to it as Starch and Sugar Addiction. From there a diet will be structured to lose excess fat without hunger, based on the nutrition needed by the body to metabolize food efficiently.

Food History

Prehistoric and ancient dates are estimates as changes were gradual over thousands of years.
Dates also vary with sources consulted. In tracing our food metabolism history, change is to be considered additive and each age includes all of the foods before. Lists of ancient foods are those in archeological records and are not intended to be all-inclusive but to provide a general overview.

Last Great Ice Age, the Pleistocene – 1 million BC to 18,000-12,000 BC. Icy tundra covered Europe and China. Climate then warms to that similar to today. The end of the Ice Age allowed agriculture to flourish in ancient civilizations and spread throughout Europe and Asia.

Early Peoples	**Old Stone Age**	**New Stone Age**
? – 60,000 BC	100,000 BC – 12,000 BC	12,000 BC–4,000 BC
Tropical to	Ice Age (Europe, China)	Village Life – More tools & Crafts
sub-tropical latitudes -	Seasonal – woods, plateaus,	*Beginnings of Agriculture*
coasts & waterways	mountains	15,000 BC - 11,000 BC

Early Peoples	Old Stone Age	New Stone Age
fruits	fruits, berries	**Agricultural Revolution**
nuts	nuts	9,000 BC – 2,000 BC
seeds	seeds	cultivated crops
leafy greens	roots	domesticated animals
roots	fish	wild wheat and barley
fish	birds	cereals
shellfish	eggs	roots, tubers
water birds	wild game such as pigs,	wild pears
eggs	goats, sheep	nuts: wild acorns, almonds,
wild game		pistachios

By 5,000 BC:
Wheat and barley cultivated in Southeastern Europe, Egypt, Turkey, Caucasus, Iran, India.
Rice and millet grown in China and Southeast Asia.

Mesopotamia

Mesopotamia cultivates the first wheat and barley from wild strains – 11,000 BC.

fish	onions	pears
mutton	garlic	apricots
pork	leeks	pomegranates
ducks	cucumbers	nuts
pigeons	cress	pistachio nuts
wheat	mustard	milk
millet	herbs	cheese
barley	lettuce	butter
barley ale	grapes	vegetable oils
(1 gal/day)	raisins	honey
chickpeas	dates	cake (flour, eggs, milk, honey)
lentils	figs	flatbread (unleavened bread)
beans	plums	
	apples	

Ancient Egypt
15,000 BC – 2,400 BC

15,000-10,000 BC	5,200 BC	3,000 – 2,400 BC
antelope	cattle	water birds & their eggs
hippos	pigs	pigeons
fish	sheep	ducks
shellfish	goats	crane
geese	cultivated emmer wheat	small uncooked,
ducks	barley	salted, pickled birds and fish
	cultivated flax (ropes,	beef
	clothing)	grapes
		figs
		berries
		onions
		milk
		cheese
		wine – red/white
		beer/ale
		flat bread
		yeast bread
		pastries
		sweet cakes

The Egyptians developed enclosed ovens for baking yeast-leavened bread from wild yeasts in 3,000 BC. Egyptian food feasts included over 40 different kinds of breads and pastries, both raised and flat, made from flour and various ingredients including honey, milk, and eggs.
The Commoner's daily food however is thought to have been a mainstay of flatbread, ale, and onions.

Ancient Greece
800 BC – 150 BC

Milk used for cheese rather than drinking.
 Breakfasts were bread and wine.
 Dinner was the large meal of the day.
 Ate with hands, few utensils.

fish	beans	asparagus
shellfish	peas	artichokes
wild game	chickpeas (garbanzo beans0	cabbage
birds	lentils	olives
chicken	grains	pears
lamb	barley, wheat	plums
beef	bread	squash
pork	cheese	leeks
pomegranates	eggs	radishes
apples	milk	turnips
	olive oil	wild celery
	vinegar	cress
	grapes	Romaine lettuce
	figs	carrots
	herbs	cucumber
	nuts	wine
	asparagus	honey mead
	nuts	beer

Ancient Rome
100 BC – 500 AD

Similar to that of Ancient Greece.
Breakfast was often bread dipped in
olive oil with wine.
Dinner was the large meal of the
day. Ate mostly with hands. Utensils
used for serving.
Milk was used for making cheese
rather than drinking.

eggs
bread
cereal
cheese

fish
shellfish
game
domestic fowl
pork
figs
dates
nuts
apples
pears
grapes
cabbage
parsnips
lettuce/salad/romaine

asparagus
onion
garlic
radishes
lentils
beans
beets
herbs
spices
cakes, pastries
    sweetened w/honey
pancakes
wine

Flour & Sugar
Age of Agriculture

Flour
Both white and brown flour are produced. White bread
is eaten mostly by the rich as it is more expensive,
taking longer to produce.

Sugarcane from India
Darius of Persia and his soldiers saw sugar cane growing
in India and called it the reed that produces honey
without bees. 510 BC. Ancients used mostly honey and
fruit sugars for sweetening.

Ancient Americas, Tropical Islands, Asia
Time frames vary. List is example only.

Indigenous meats, game, fish, birds,
seafood.
maize/corn
tortilla/taco
tamale
pineapple
papaya
banana
avocado
tomatoes
cacao
coffee

yams
sweet potatoes
potatoes
grapefruit
bell peppers
chili peppers
winter & summer squash
pumpkin
beans-pinto, red, black
vanilla bean
peanuts

tea
noodles
rice
millet
soy sauce
tofu
sesame seeds/oil
bamboo shoots
sake/rice wine
herbs
spices

European Medieval Food
1100 – 1500 AD

Increased emphasis on meat and bread as foundation foods with fewer fruits and vegetables available in the colder climates.

beef
pork
lamb
fish
birds

barley bread, cereal
barley ale
French wine
cheese
milk
eggs
salted and preserved for winter
  fish, beef, pork

cabbage
leeks
spinach
parsley
onions
garlic
honey
sugar, spices – imported

Industrial Revolution
1760 – 2000 AD

Increasing mass production of foods
Refined flours
Refined white sugar from
  sugar beets and sugar cane

1700's – Wheat replaces rye and barley as primary grain in Europe when sturdier wheat is developed for the colder climate

refined
processed
treated
cloned, hybrid
frozen, boxed, canned,
  shaped, formed,
  wrapped
.

chemicals
artificial flavors, colors
preservatives
starchy fillers
corn syrup
salt, excessive
sugar, excessive
hydrogenated fats

BREAD & GRAIN PRODUCTS
Rated Best to Worst for Metabolic Compatibility
Determined by Use in History as Natural Foods

Best: Least Fat Effect

Rating	Product Today	Reason
1	Whole grain cereals, to cook. Whole wheat, barley, flax, brown rice, rye, oatmeal.	Stone Age – 50,000 BC to 12,000 BC Gathered Seeds including wild wheat and barley. Wheat was emmer wheat, a crude wild wheat gathered in Mediterranean areas. Wild rice in Asia. Whole grain natural nutrients. Often mixed with vegetable soups and sometimes eaten mixed with water or milk as a drinkable cereal or gruel.
2	Whole grain flatbreads and pastas without leavening. Pita, tortillas, pasta (no baking powder, baking soda, preservatives, trans fats, or other additives).	Emmer wheat and barley are cultivated into domestic strains. 11,000 BC. Beginnings of Agricultural Revolution. First breads are ground, mixed with water or fruit juice and cooked. Whole grain natural nutrients.
3	Yeast leavened bread, whole wheat. Yeast is ancient and compatible. Home baked or fresh bakery bread without preservatives or additives. Whole wheat french bread.	3,000 BC: Egyptians bake yeast breads from wild yeasts. Northern Europeans and those in British Isles also baked bread from wild yeast very early.
4	Yeast leavened bread, white, enriched. Includes french bread and pizza crust. Without preservatives or additives. Pasta, white, enriched, nonleavened, usually preferred with white flour.	Both dark and light breads are eaten, with the rich preferring white, but more expensive to produce. White has fewer nutrients with wheat germ and seed coat removed. Romans. 100 BC – 500 AD

5	Pastry without leavening. Pie crust	Pastry is unleavened flour product but usually high in fats and sugar and usually made with less-nutritious white flour.
6	Pastry, yeast-leavened. Donuts, rolls, maple bars, etc. Fresh baked, no preservatives.	Yeast leavening is metabolic complement. However, today's fat and high refined sugar content require restraint.

Worst: Most Fat Effect

7	Tea breads, biscuits, scones, cookies, cake donuts, cakes, pancakes leavened with chemical baking powder and baking soda.	Baking powder and baking soda are relatively new leavening agents, the products of the manufacturing age since 1800s. Leavened with eggs okay. Home baked borderline okay. Usually high sugar and fat content.
8	Off the shelf flour products: cookies, cakes, muffins, crackers, donuts, rolls, bread, chips, cereals. Manufactured, processed, preserved.	Industrial. Last 200 years. Packed with artificial ingredients.

KA

3

Fat Melt Dynamic

So far we have established the foundation of our diet to be a world of foods natural to metabolism. However, this is not enough. A plan of action is needed, a plan of action that will melt away excess fat with a balance of foods needed by the body, without hardship and hunger, a necessity for successful dieting and weight control. However, the first step is to stop the process that is causing the wrong choices in food.

Stop Starch & Sugar Addiction – SSSA

Plain and simple, this is an addiction to flour and sugar products. The effects are the need to constantly eat more without satisfaction, causing excess fat buildup. If we look at excess fat as a picture of the foods that are eaten, what do we see? Certainly not fruits and vegetables. We see an endless variety of cake, cookies, chips, crackers, fast food, convenience foods, and rich sweets, all refined white flour and refined white sugar foods, manufactured for profit. Why these foods are so addictive may be due to multiple factors. One is that refined white sugar is not a natural food because it is highly concentrated from the natural sugar cane or the sugar beet from which it is made. In the process, nutrients are extracted in the juices, leaving little nutrition for metabolism and lots of addiction. In white flour, the wheat germ and the wheat bran of the whole wheat are discarded along with needed nutrition. The reason these nutrients are needed is because the body needs the metabolic materials, the vitamins and minerals, to which it has adapted over thousands of years, as discussed in the last chapter. Some people's bodies may also be more vulnerable to this addiction.

Additionally, with manufacturing, these flour and sugar products have all kinds of additional ingredients alien to the body of the ages, designed for long shelf life with cheap thrills to the taste buds. The cheap thrills are excessive salt, fats, artificial flavors, syrups and sugars. Added for profit are all kinds of starchy fillers and preservatives. For eye appeal, artificial colors are added along with attractive packaging. The food value of these foods is negative as the body tries to metabolize the strange ingredients and seems to want more food, searching for more nutrients to help metabolize the ones it has.

Therefore, the first step is to realize these foods are addictive for whatever reason and to give them up as LTN or Little to No eating while losing excess fat. This allows the body to rest from the onslaught and sets it up for the nutrition it needs. The first stages of the diet therefore restrict these types of flour and sugar products. Not all manufactured products are excluded however. For example, artificial sweeteners are helpful in the first stages of the diet in restricting refined white sugar.

However, starch and sugar are just other words for carbohydrates. Carbohydrate foods have thousands of starch molecules which are broken up into different kinds of sugars in the body. All carbohydrates are starch and sugar. The distinction is between *natural* carbohydrates and *natural* sugars and *manufactured* food carbohydrates. The body needs the *natural* carbohydrates, full of nutrition and vitamins and minerals. The natural carbs and sugars are not fattening nor do they cause addiction. Therefore, the diet, to stop flour and sugar addiction, in the first few days of the menus, will replace the starch and sugar in refined flour and refined sugar with natural fruit sugars and milk sugars. Once these addictive flours and sugars are restricted, dieters look forward to the enjoyment of natural fruits and vegetables, chosen from a huge variety of foods.

Natural Carbohydrates

In stopping the starch and sugar addiction, food is not given up but only replaced. The replacement food is natural carbohydrates. Carbohydrates are all the foods that are not a protein or a fat. Food is categorized according to how it is digested by the body and carbohydrates become sugars, sugars needed by the body. As pointed out, natural carbohydrates are not fattening because they contain all the nutrients needed for metabolism. Therefore, the diet includes abundant carbohydrate foods.

Fruits and vegetables have essential vitamins and minerals needed by the body for metabolism. For this reason, they need to be thought of as metabolism tuners that make metabolic processes burn brightly, directly dissolving excess fat stores. The fruits need to be appealingly sweet and juicy and liberally enjoyed, such as eating as much as wanted, especially when giving up starch and sugar addiction. Peelings, skins, and seeds should be sampled. These are part of metabolic heritage.

Steamed cooked vegetables are an important part of the diet as they add up to more total vegetables and more choices than raw vegetables alone. Vegetables too are full of vitamins and minerals and natural sugars that melt away excess fat. The more vegetables eaten, the better fat can be metabolized.

Also included are the heavy duty carbs like rice, beans, and potatoes. These are great satisfactions that help prevent hunger. As natural carbs with natural nutrients, they are not fattening. Other major carbohydrate foods, such as bread, grains, and pasta were discussed in the last chapter.

In addition, natural sugars such as honey, raw unrefined sugar, and natural maple syrups are metabolically friendly and do not cause addiction or weight gain.

High Protein

Protein gets special attention in the diet because it is the most difficult food category to maintain in adequate amounts. Daily protein intake needs to be around one half normal, or target, body weight. For example, a person that should weigh 190 pounds needs around 80 grams of protein a day. Protein is a very important nutrient, needed for maintenance and repair for every cell in the body. While even plant foods have protein, they are not complete proteins. Beans are high in protein but are not complete proteins and need other foods, such as rice, corn, or meat to balance out the needed amounts. Complete proteins are the foods that supply the eight or nine missing proteins or amino acids that the body cannot produce for itself. These need to be supplied daily. These are the EAAs or essential amino acids. Complete protein foods are meat type foods such as fish, shellfish, poultry, beef, and pork. Dairy foods also have complete protein. Soybeans are the primary plant regarded as a complete protein food.

In the diet, dairy foods are used as a convenient, economical way to boost protein levels throughout the day. This includes yogurt, cottage cheese, milk, and protein drinks made with soy or whey. Whey is a byproduct of cheese making and is high in protein. Eggs are also a complete protein food full of nutrients.

With the increased interest in yogurt, many more choices are now available. Not only is yogurt a complete protein, it contains healthy bacteria, such as *lactobacillus acidophilus*, which are very beneficial to the intestinal system. The names of these bacteria are usually listed on the container for quality yogurt, abbreviated because they are very long. These bacteria may also help boost the synthesis of B complex vitamins in the body. B complex vitamins are powerhouses that boost all kinds of metabolic processes. In addition yogurt, along with the other dairy products, contains calcium and magnesium, which contribute to the feelings of peace and tranquility on the diet.

However, yogurt packed with refined sugar is to be avoided. Lowfat, artificially flavored and sweetened yogurt, especially in the first phases of the diet, when stopping starch and sugar addiction, is recommended. This is referred to as diet yogurt, around 100 calories. The LYD (Love Your Diet) yogurt is all natural yogurt, with no added sugar, mixed with a few tablespoons of the diet yogurt for flavor. See the menu explanations.

The diet is structured to maintain protein levels throughout the day, beginning with breakfast, which should contain 15 to 20 grams protein, hunger snacks with around 10 grams protein each, and another 20 grams each for lunch and dinner. This totals around 70 to 80 grams protein for the day. Adequate protein helps burn fat, build muscle, prevent hunger and fatigue, and maintain skin tone during dieting.

Lowfat, rather than nonfat, dairy products are recommended because the body needs some fats to metabolize fat soluble vitamins A, D, E, and K. Fats and oils are also healthy for skin, hair, and tissue. However, at 100 calories per tablespoon, it makes sense to keep fats and oils to a minimum when reducing.

No Hunger

This is not a hunger diet. Hunger is to be avoided because it is counter productive and miserable. When eating the right foods, fat melts away without hunger. In addition, the body feels stress when hungry as though surviving a famine and will fight against fat loss. The body must feel it is safe to "let go" of the excess fat. Therefore hunger is to be avoided. Three levels of hunger can be identified:

Level 1 Hunger: This is the first stages of hunger felt as gentle reminders that food will be needed soon. Level 1 hunger can be forgotten for small amounts of time.

Level 2 Hunger: This is the next stage of hunger, which is constant and does not go away.

Level 3 Hunger: Level 3 hunger is intense. This is the stage where the body feels it must have food or be in danger of starvation. It wants food immediately. Many traditional diet plans require enduring level 3 hunger, which only willpower can sustain and then only for so long. The diet is usually broken by the strongest willed, who then go for the fattest food they can find. At level 3 hunger, the dieter risks eating any food available. Level 3 hunger is to be avoided.

On this diet, eating at Level 1 hunger keeps the body tuned to burning fat without the feeling of starvation while avoiding the discomfort and misery of deprivation.

Maximum Calories

Yes, calories need to be counted on this diet but it is different. It is not a hunger inducing restricted calorie diet. Rather, the maximum calories for current weight is used. This is accomplished by multiplying 12 times the current weight. The result is the amount of calories being used. For example, for a person weighing 200 pounds, 12 times that weight would be 2400 calories, the upper limit to strive for in calories for the day. As the body gets the nutritious foods it needs, rather than the fat producing foods, it begins to reduce fat stores on its own, without calorie reduction. The 12 factor represents a moderately active lifestyle, sitting at computers or a desk, or watching TV part of the day.

It is probably a huge disservice for traditional and trendy diet plans to not count calories. Without counting calories, dieters are kept in the dark for options, limited to only that particular diet. Food has to be unnecessarily restricted to get results and hunger is a constant companion. By counting calories and weighing in every morning, before eating and drinking, the dieter can keep track of how the diet is working and see immediately if straying from the diet causes weight gain.

The *Love Your Diet Calorie Counter, Maximum Calories: The Goldilocks Paradigm* is available on Amazon or the website at *www.loveyourdietseries.com* and makes calorie counting easy. Two calorie amounts are given: first, for a small amount of the food which can easily be multiplied times the amount eaten and secondly, another amount for an average serving. Calorie counting increases knowledge about foods, helps in reading food labels, and provides the numbers to track what is actually being eaten.

Next, are the menus that bring together all of the above fat melting dynamics: stopping starch and sugar addiction, replacing bad carbohydrates with natural carbohydrates, maintaining high protein levels, preventing hunger, and eating maximum calories. The menus also add table wine, bread, and pasta on the principles outlined in Chapter 2, *Code of the Ancient Harvest*, as foods compatible with metabolism. Additionally, these are foods and beverages that not only add to dieting pleasure but to the artistry of dining. The menus also provide for the essential balance and variety of foods needed to meet the nutritional needs of the body. The body does not need just one or two foods, but a spectrum of foods.

What happens if the dieter simply adds the healthy foods, more fruits and vegetables and more protein, while still eating the addictive starch and sugar LTN foods? Then it is not the diet and it will not work to reduce excess fat. The diet depends on *replacing* the starch and sugar offenders, not adding to them. It is possible to lose weight on the starch and sugar fast fat foods only if calories are drastically and miserably reduced to a level of constant hunger. On the other hand, with this diet, these foods can be eaten occasionally without harm. Again, the scale and daily weigh-ins are the measure. When eating the delicious food on this diet, these other foods lose their attraction.

The basic wine primer for the menus is a very generalized list for the person who does not have a lot of experience with different kinds of wine. The value of wine is that it adds a feeling of luxury to a meal and decreases any feelings of deprivation. Wine complements food, adding to its flavor and enjoyment. A glass of wine with fresh fruits and vegetables while preparing dinner, then with dinner, makes food a feast.

Knowledge of wines can be very complex and expensive, requiring study and experience. In general, the more expensive the wine, the better. Good wines have more character, depth, and complexity, changing with different foods. Good wine is an art worthy of exploration. However, inexpensive, moderately priced table wines can be used daily, according to personal preference and budget. A good rule however is to only have wine with food and not by itself. Otherwise, it goes to the head quite fast on an empty stomach. Alcohol can be similar to sugar in addictive qualities. Drinking only with food prevents reliance on alcohol. Polishing off a meal with something sweet such as fruit and honey or 70% and above cacao chocolate, stops any felt need for more wine. Measuring out the amount to drink ahead of time and counting the calories is also helpful.

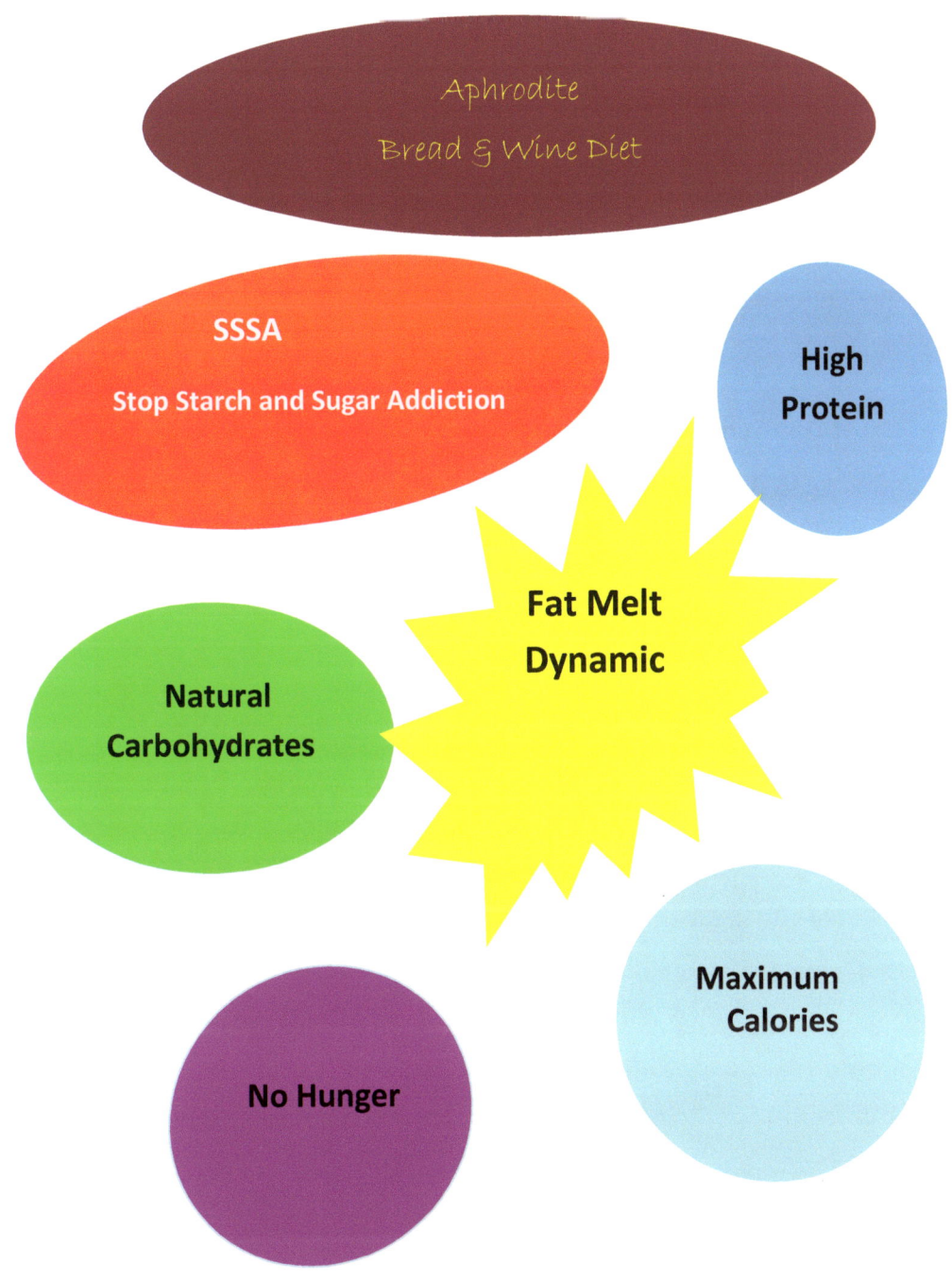

4

Aphrodite Bread & Wine Diet Menus

Contents

Menu Terms and Definitions

SSSA   Stop Starch & Sugar Addiction
                    The first 3 days of the diet replaces processed manufactured starch and sugar and
                    all flour and refined sugar with fruit sugars, milk sugars, and generous natural carbs.

LTN   Little To No, Little To None, Foods

Level 1 Hunger   The beginning twinges of hunger

Anytime   Water
Beverages   Coffee
                    Flavorings: No artificial creamers. Use natural cream, half & half, lowfat milk,
                    or powdered milk. Sweeten with raw sugar, demerara sugar, or honey.
                  Tea
                    Flavor with milk, raw sugar, demerara sugar. honey, lemon, if needed.
                  Diet Sugar Free Soda
                    (exception: children should have instead lowfat milk, all natural fruit juice, water,
                    or naturally flavored water)
                  Cranberry Water
                    1 C water with 2 T to 1/4C all natural, concentrated cranberry juice
                  Lemon Water
                    1 C water with 1 to 2 t lemon juice

Diet Yogurt   Avoid yogurt with added sugar (180-250 calories per 8 oz). Nonfat & lowfat
                  may still have lots of sugar added. Read labels.
                  Diet yogurt to use is lowfat, artificially sweetened and flavored (100-120
                  calories per 8 oz) Read labels.

All Natural   Natural yogurt containing live bacteria and no added sugar beyond milk
Yogurt , Lowfat   sugars.
                    .

LYD Yogurt   Love Your Diet Yogurt: Mix 2T to 1/4C lowfat, flavored, diet yogurt (above)
                  with 8 oz all natural yogurt, above. (Note: Organic does not necessarily
                  mean no added sugar. Read labels.)

C   Cup or 8 oz cup measure
oz   ounce
T   Tablespoon
t   teaspoon
lb   pound

Table Wine Basics

Wine can be a complex study of taste, grapes, year, weather, age, climate, soil, location, methods of production, vineyard, etc. Therefore, this is only an outline. Go on internet for more information or consult articles and books on wine. Generally, the more expensive the better the wine (more depth and complexity), but many excellent affordable wines are available. Dry wines (not sweet) in general are best with food as they complement rather than drown the taste of the food. Currently, any glass will do and individual taste determines what wine goes with what food. In general however, red wines go with more robust tasting food (steak, pasta) and white with more light and delicate food (fish, poultry). A wine that is a good complement to a food enhances the flavor of the food and takes on complexities of its own depending on the accompanying food (usually a characteristic of more expensive wines). The name of the wine is based on the primary type of grape used.

Name	Taste	Food
Reds		
Cabernet Sauvignon *Ca ber nay'* *Sow veen yon'*	dry, full bodied	beef, steak, pork, pasta, cheese, bread, fruit, chocolate
Merlot *Mer low'*	dry, light bodied	similar to cabernet sauvignon but lighter
Pinot Noir *Pe'no nwahr*	dry, fruity, medium to full bodied	red meats, cheese, fruit, bread
French designations Bordeaux *Bor doe' or claret*	dry, light, fruity, full bodied, delicate	red meats, cheese, fruit, bread
Burgundy *(Bur' gun dee)*	burgundy heavier and more full bodied than bordeaux	
Beaujolais *Bow sjo lay'*	light, fruity, best when young	cheese, fruit, red meats
Italian Chianti *Key on'tey*	dry, medium bodied	tomato sauce pasta, cheese, bread
Whites Chardonay *shar do nay'*	dry, fruity, full body	fish, shellfish, poultry
Rhine *rine,* Moselle *mo zel'*	dry, light body	poultry, fish, cheese
Chablis *sha blee'*	dry, light, fruity	poultry, cheese, fruit
Sauvignon Blanc *So'veen yo blawnc'*	medium dry, light, fruity	fish, poultry, cheese, fruit
Rose (some red skins of grapes color the wine) *Ro zay'*	lightly sweet to sweet	fruit, cheese
Champagne *Sham payne'*	bubbly, dry to sweet driest is brut (bru)	Dry accompanies appetizers and dinner while sweeter varieties best with dessert. *KA*

Aphrodite Bread & Wine Diet
High Protein Menu Model

Protein: Count major proteins only (meat, dairy). Protein amounts listed in *Love Your Diet Calorie Counters*. Daily grams of complete protein need to be near ½ of desired weight. Example: normal target weight of 150 lbs =   75 grams protein daily.

Dairy: average protein per 8 oz = 8-10 grams protein. Meats: average per 4 oz serving = 20-30 grams protein.
 See Chapter 6 – High Protein.

Breakfast 15-20 grams protein	**Protein food and whole grain cereal with fruit** ¼ C natural, to-cook rolled oats cereal with fresh diced apple, raw sugar, and ½ C lowfat milk. ½ C milk = 4 grams protein **AND** 1 whole large egg = 6 grams protein (yolk = 2.7 grams protein, white = 3.6 grams protein) **AND/OR** any of the following (fresh raw fruit optional): ½ C – 1C 1% Cottage cheese: ½ C = 14 grams protein; 1C = 28 grams protein. High protein nutrition drink: 1T = 7 grams protein plus milk @ 8 grams protein = 15grams protein. See label. 1C Diet Yogurt or LYD Yogurt : 6-11 grams protein
Level 1 Hunger Snacks 10+ grams protein	**Protein food plus fruit and/or vegetables at first feelings of hunger** Yogurt Cottage cheese Vegetable juice Fruit - fresh, raw Vegetables – fresh, raw Nutrition or Diet Drink
Lunch 20+ grams protein	**Meat (Deli chicken or Fish)** Sometimes: Chicken & Jo-Jos or Fish & Chips 4 oz chicken thigh, batter-dipped = 25 grams protein. 4 oz fish, battered fillet, as fish and chips, 16 grams protein. **Vegetables – raw or cooked and/or green salad** **OR** Continue Hunger Snacks
Level 1 Hunger Snacks 10+ grams protein	Same as morning Yogurt Vegetables, fruit – raw, fresh
While Preparing Dinner	**Raw, fresh vegetables and/or fruit** Sliced avocado, tomato, cucumber , raw finger food with or without low-cal

dressing dip
Fruit – fresh, raw, melons, berries, grapes
Table Wine or Anytime Beverage

Dinner
20-30+ grams protein

Protein, Vegetables
Meat (fish, chicken, other) lightly fried or sautéed in olive oil and garlic.
Potato - large, microwaved, served with sour cream **OR**
1 C Rice with tamari soy sauce **OR** 1 large, 10 oz Sweet Potato **OR** Yam with butter or margarine **OR** 1 C Beans
1-2 C Vegetables – cooked, served with sour cream, butter, or low-cal margarine
Table Wine – if wanted

Dessert

Fresh fruit with chocolate sauce and whipped topping **OR**
Pudding, instant, non-sugar, lowfat **OR**
Ice Cream, no sugar added, with fruit and/or chocolate sauce

Anytime Snacks

Raw seeds & nuts (in shell, no oil added) & raw, fresh fruit

KA

Aphrodite Bread & Wine Diet
SSSA – Stop Starch & Sugar Addiction
Starter Menu – Day 1

Breakfast
1 C lowfat cottage cheese with fresh apricots

Level 1 Hunger Snack - Morning
1 – 2 C Diet or LYD Yogurt with fresh blueberries
1 – 2 C grapes, red or black, seeded - as much as wanted

Lunch
Green salad with garbanzo beans & grated cheese
Red or black grapes – as much wanted

Level 1 Hunger Snack - Afternoon
Same as morning

Before Dinner Appetizer
Sliced cucumbers, tomatoes, radishes
4 oz chardonnay

Dinner
4 - 6 oz salmon fillet, wild caught
1 C rice with tamari soy sauce
1 C steamed asparagus with 1 T sour cream
4 oz chardonnay

Dessert
Banana Split
1 banana
2 T chocolate sauce
2 T whipped topping
1 T peanuts

After Dinner Hunger Snack
Repeat dessert or
Nibblers - nuts, seeds, dried fruit

KA

Aphrodite Bread & Wine Diet

SSSA – Stop Starch & Sugar Addiction
Starter Menu – Day 2

Breakfast
3 egg omelet or 1 whole egg and 3 whites

Level 1 Hunger Snack - Morning
1 – 2 C Diet or Yogurt
1 – 2 C sweet cherries - as much as wanted

Lunch
2 – 3 pieces deli chicken with batter
4 – 6 oz potato wedges or jo-jos with thousand island dip

Level 1 Hunger Snack - Afternoon
Same as morning

Before Dinner Appetizer
Sliced avocado, tomato, cucumber
4 oz cabernet sauvignon or pinot noir

Dinner
4 – 6 oz ribeye steak
1 slice French garlic bread, bakery fresh, no preservatives
10 oz baked potato with 1 T sour cream and chopped chives or green onion
1 C steamed mustard greens and spinach with 1 T sour cream
4 oz cabernet or pinot noir

Dessert
1 C no sugar added ice cream
2 T chocolate sauce
2 T whipped topping

After Dinner Hunger Snack
Repeat dessert or
Nibblers - nuts, seeds, dried fruit

KA

Aphrodite Bread & Wine Diet

SSSA – Stop Starch & Sugar Addiction
Starter Menu – Day 3

Breakfast
1 C lowfat cottage cheese

Level 1 Hunger Snack - Morning

1 – 2 C Diet or Yogurt
1 – 2 C strawberries - as much as wanted

Lunch
2 – 3 oz tuna on green salad

Level 1 Hunger Snack - Afternoon
Same as morning

Before Dinner Appetizer
Vegetables – cucumber, sweet pepper
4 oz chardonnay

Dinner

6 – 8 oz shrimp, 26-30 per lb. frozen or fresh, tail on, shelled, cleaned
Sautéed in olive oil, garlic, sweet pepper, green onion
1 C rice with 1 T tamari soy sauce
1 C steamed broccoli with 1 T sour cream
4 oz chardonnay

Dessert
½ C strawberries
1 T chocolate sauce
1 T whipped topping

After Dinner Hunger Snack
Repeat dessert or
Nibblers - nuts, seeds, fruit

KA

Aphrodite Bread & Wine Diet

Menu – Day 4

Menu Terms and Definitions at beginning of chapter.

Breakfast
1 C oatmeal
½ C yogurt with fresh blueberries
1 boiled egg with 1 t butter and paprika

Level 1 Hunger Snack - Morning
1 C Yogurt

Lunch
1 – 2 C yogurt
Green salad

Level 1 Hunger Snack - Afternoon
Same as morning

Before Dinner Appetizer
Fruit – grapes, sliced apple
4 oz chablis or sauvignon blanc

Dinner

2 – 3 boneless chicken thighs simmered with garlic, lemon and rosemary
10 oz sweet potato or yam with 1 T butter or margarine
1 C steamed green beans and carrots with 1 T sour cream
4 oz chablis

Dessert
Apple Delight
1 sliced apple with 1 t demerara sugar warmed in microwave
1 T cream or ½ C no-sugar-added vanilla ice cream

After Dinner Hunger Snack
Repeat dessert

KA

Aphrodite Bread & Wine Diet

Menu – Day 5
Menu Terms and Definitions at beginning of chapter.

Breakfast
1 C lowfat cottage cheese
2 slices whole wheat toast, bakery fresh, no preservatives

Level 1 Hunger Snack - Morning
Apple, raisins, walnuts or pecans

Lunch
Restaurant fish and chips (potatoes, not potato chips)
Green salad

Level 1 Hunger Snack - Afternoon
Same as morning

Before Dinner Appetizer
Grapes, olives
1 slice bakery fresh French bread with hummus spread
4 oz Italian Chianti

Dinner
1 – 2 C spaghetti with mushroom sauce, homemade, topped with 1-2 T parmesan
1 – 2 slices French bread with olive oil, butter, chopped garlic
Green salad with lowcal Italian dressing
4 oz Italian Chianti

Dessert
Peaches and Cream
1 - 2 fresh peaches, sliced, warmed with 1 t demerara sugar
2 T cream or half and half

After Dinner Hunger Snack
Repeat dessert

KA

Aphrodite Bread & Wine Diet

Menu – Day 6
Menu Terms and Definitions at beginning of chapter.

Breakfast
1 C oatmeal
1 slice whole wheat toast, bakery fresh, no preservatives
1 C LYD yogurt with fresh blueberries

Level 1 Hunger Snack - Morning
Sunflower seeds and peanuts

Lunch
1 – 2 C yogurt
Green salad

Level 1 Hunger Snack - Afternoon
Same as morning

Before Dinner Appetizer
Apple with 1 oz cheese
1 slice French bread with olive oil butter and chopped garlic
4 oz chardonnay

Dinner
3 – 4 oz cod fillet simmered in olive oil, lemon, garlic, thyme
1 C rice with tamari soy sauce
Steamed cabbage wedge with carrots with 1 T sour cream
4 oz chardonnay

Dessert
Banana Split
Sliced banana
1 C no sugar added ice cream
1 T whipped topping or whipped cream

After Dinner Hunger Snack
Repeat dessert

KA

Aphrodite Bread & Wine Diet

Menu – Day 7

Menu Terms and Definitions at beginning of chapter.

Breakfast
1 C oatmeal
1 slice whole wheat toast, bakery fresh, no preservatives
1 egg boiled with 1 t butter and sprinkled with paprika

Level 1 Hunger Snack - Morning
Sliced tomatoes and cucumbers

Lunch
1 – 2 C yogurt
Green salad

Level 1 Hunger Snack - Afternoon
Same as morning

Before Dinner Appetizer
Sliced red and yellow sweet pepper, black olives
1 slice French bread with olive oil butter and chopped garlic
4 oz chablis, chardonnay, or sauvignon blanc

Dinner
1 Cornish game hen, stuffed with rice, roasted with garlic, lemon, rosemary
1 C rice with tamari soy sauce
Steamed fresh green beans with 1 T sour cream
4 oz dry white wine as above

Dessert
1 slice no sugar added apple pie
½ C no sugar added vanilla ice cream

After Dinner Hunger Snack
Repeat dessert

KA

Menu Substitutions
& Protein Amounts
Anytime Beverages listed in *Menu Terms and Definitions* at beginning of chapter

Breakfast - Choose food equal to 15-20 grams (gr) protein

1 large egg – 6 gr protein	1 C cottage cheese – 28-30 gr protein	Fruits, raw, fresh
3 eggs – 18 gr protein	1 C Diet or LYD Yogurt – 8-11 gr protein	Whole wheat toast
1 egg yolk – 2.7 gr protein	1 C High Protein Drink – 12-15 gr	To-cook oatmeal
1 egg white – 3.6 gr protein	4 oz meat, poultry, fish -- 25 gr protein	Natural fruit juice
	1 C lowfat milk – 8 gr protein	

Morning Hunger Snacks - Choose food equal to 8-10 grams protein

Protein foods same as breakfast	Fruit – raw, fresh, juicy	Seeds, nuts
	Vegetables – raw, fresh, sliced	Dried fruit

Lunch – Choose food equal to at least 8-10 grams protein

Protein foods same as breakfast	4 oz poultry, meat, seafood – 25 gr protein	Vegetables/salad
Potatoes – wedge or baked	Flatbread, pita	Fruit, raw, fresh
Beans, rice	Tortillas	Hunger snacks

Afternoon Hunger Snacks – Choose food equal to 8-10 grams protein
Same as morning hunger snacks. Eat at Level 1 Hunger

Before Dinner Appetizers – Curb appetite while preparing dinner

Hummus	Vegetables, raw – sweet peppers,	Fruits, fresh, raw
French bread, bakery fresh	olives, celery, radishes, cucumbers,	melons, peaches,
Whole wheat bread, bakery	tomatoes,	Berries, apple,
	See fruits and vegetables lists in *Foods to Eat*	

Dinner – Choose food equal to 20+ grams protein

Natural "heavy-duty" carbs:	Poultry, seafood, lean meat	Vegetables - cooked
potatoes, rice, beans, yams,	4 Oz – average 25 gr protein	See *Foods to Eat*
sweet potatoes	French bread, bakery fresh	

Desserts – Control (LTN) refined white sugar and manufactured foods

Artificially-sweetened	Fruits, raw, fresh	Natural cream
Ice cream, pies, pudding, gelatin	Raw honey and demerera sugar	Whipped topping
Sometimes – yeast donuts	Chocolate sauce	See *Foods to Eat*

After Dinner Snack
Satisfy any hunger with Snacks and Nibblers listed in Foods to Eat or repeat dessert.

KA

Aphrodite Bread & Wine Diet
Foods to Eat

Protein Foods
Poultry – Chicken, Turkey, Duck
Fish – All Varieties, fresh, frozen
Shellfish – Shrimp, Prawns, Lobster, Oysters, Scallops, Crab
Meat – Beef, Pork (lean), Wild Game (deer, elk), Buffalo
Dairy Products
Milk – 1%
Cottage Cheese - 1%
Yogurt – Diet Lowfat, Artificially-Sweetened – 100 calories
Yogurt --LYD -Love Your Diet Yogurt – All natural, no added
    sugar yogurt mixed with 2T – ¼ C Diet Yogurt- 150 calories
Eggs - Fresh, Low Cholesterol
Nutrition Drinks - Flavored, whey, soy protein

Fruit - All Varieties, Fresh, Raw

Vegetables - All Varieties, Fresh, Raw or Cooked

Potatoes (Tubers)
White Potatoes
Sweet Potatoes
Yams

Grains
Rice - Natural, Brown or White, To-cook, Non-instant
Cereal - Natural Whole-grain, To-cook
Oatmeal
Whole Wheat
Mixed Grain

Beans (Legumes), Home-cooked, all varieties

Sweeteners
Sugar - Raw, Unrefined
Demerera Sugar – type of raw sugar
Turbinado Sugar – type of raw sugar
Honey
Natural Maple Syrup

Anytime Beverages
Water
Coffee
Tea
Diet Soda
Milk – Lowfat
Cranberry juice water
Lemon juice water

Sometimes Beverages
Wine
Beer

Condiments
Sour Cream
Soy Sauce
Cocktail Sauce
Lemon Juice - fresh
Sauces for Meat
Herbs, Spices

Desserts
Fruit
Pudding, Gelatin - Non-sugar
Whipped Topping
Chocolate Sauce
Cream
Honey
Ice Cream - No Sugar Added
70%+ Cacao Chocolate bar

Fats, Oils
Olive Oil – cold press, first press
Butter
Canola Oil & Canola Margarine
Butter & Yogurt Margarine

Snacks & Nibblers
Nuts, Seeds
Fruits, Vegetables
Popcorn – Air-popped
Raisins, Dried Fruit

Sometimes Foods (every 4 to 7 days)
Bakery Bread - Yeast Leavened - French, Italian, Wh. Wheat
Pasta & Sauce - Homemade Meals
Breads - Unleavened - Pita, Tortillas, Tacos
Pancakes - Whole Wheat w/Fruit & Natural Maple Syrup
Pizza
Submarine Sandwiches – Bakery Loaf Bread
    homemade or Fast Food Lean- Turkey, Lean Ham, vegetables
Batter-dipped in Tempura Flour, Fried in Olive Oil - Shrimp,
    Oysters, Onions, Vegetables

Go Easy Foods
Sweeteners
Cereals
Chocolate Sauce
Chocolate bar
Cream
Ice Cream
Cheese
Breaded, Batter-dipped
Beer
Wine
Butter
Oils
Fats
Salt
Pasta
Breads

Supplements
Vitamin-Mineral Tablet
Brewer's Yeast
High Protein Drink

KA

Aphrodite Bread & Wine Diet
What Not to Eat – The LTN (Little to No) Foods

FOOD/INGREDIENT	Type	Average Calories /Amount
Bagels	All varieties.	80/oz
Biscuits	Made with flour, baking powder.	100/oz
Biscuits	Made from refrigerated dough.	90/oz
Breads	Packaged and preserved.	70-80/oz
Breads, Bakery – Sometimes Food	OK: Fresh, yeast-leavened, no preservatives or additives.	80/oz
Brownies	Regular or lowfat.	100/oz
Cakes	All varieties.	105/oz
Candy & candy bars	All varieties.	Various
Canned foods	Soup, beans, pasta. Exceptions: vegetables & fruit in natural juices.	Various
Carbonated sodas	Sweetened with sugar syrups. High sugar count.	150/12 oz 13 per oz
Cereals	Ready-to-eat. Sugars, additives.	80-120/oz
Chips	Tortilla, nacho, corn, potato.	140-150/oz
Cookies	All varieties.	100/oz
Corn syrup products	Added as sweetener to prepared foods.	Various
Crackers	All varieties-cheese, saltine, graham, wheat, rye.	120-140/oz
English muffins	All varieties.	65/oz
Flour – Sometimes Food	Flour and flour products. Gluten additives for fillers.	Various
Food Additives	Starches - flour, gluten, cornstarch, sugar, corn syrup. Artificial colors and flavorings. Preservatives.	Various
French toast	All varieties.	75/oz
Frozen dinners	All varieties. Artificially flavored. Flour & thickeners. High salt.	25-200/oz
Frozen foods	All varieties. Artificially sweetened and flavored. Flour & thickeners. High salt. Exceptions: Fish, batter-coated fish, vegetables, fruit--natural, non-sweetened. Whipped topping. Meatless patties. Soy and vegetable burgers.	Various
Gravies	All varieties.	30-100/1/4 C
Hot dogs & frankfurters	All varieties. Preservatives.	140/each

Ice cream	Fully sweetened with sugars and syrups. High sugar count. Chemical preservatives & flavors. Exceptions: all natural, no sugar added, artificial sweetener OK, regular or lowfat OK.	280/8 oz cup 35 per oz
Juice Drinks	Added water, flavorings, sugar, corn syrup, high sugar count	115/8 oz 14 per oz
Liquors	Gin, vodka, rum, whiskey.	100/1.5 oz
Luncheon meat	Bologna, salami, beef, pork, chicken, turkey. Preservatives.	60-90/oz
Margarines & shortenings	High in trans fats or hydrogenated oils.	75-115/T
Meats, preserved, cured	All varieties. Luncheon meat, sausage, ham, hot dogs, bacon.	100/oz
Milk shakes	Fully sweetened with sugars and syrups. Artificial flavors.	350/10 oz 35 per oz
Muffins	All varieties.	80-85/oz
Packaged foods & dinners Dry, canned, frozen	Macaroni, rice, spaghetti, pudding. Additives. Exception: Artificially sweetened puddings and gelatin desserts for dieting.	Various
Pancakes/waffles – Sometimes Food	All varieties. Exception: homemade once a week.	40-80/oz
Pasta – Sometimes Food	All varieties. Exception: OK every 4 -7 days.	25/oz
Pastries	All varieties-doughnuts, Danish, éclairs, cinnamon rolls, toaster pastries.	105-120/oz
Pies	All varieties. Exception: No sugar added fruit OK once a week.	75/oz
Potato chips	All varieties.	150/oz
Pretzels	All varieties.	110/oz
Rolls	Dinner rolls.	85/oz
Rolls	Hot Dog & hamburger.	80/oz
Sausages.	Salami, pork, beef, dry.	120/oz
Snack cakes	Packaged, crème-filled	105/oz
Soup	All prepared varieties. Additives. High salt.	100-200/oz
Spaghetti – Sometimes Food	All varieties. Exception: OK every 4-7 days, homemade.	25/oz
Syrup	Corn syrup. Imitation maple and artificial flavorings.	60/T
Tacos, Tortillas, Pita – Sometimes Foods	OK every 4-7 days.	Various.
Yogurts	Sweetened with sugar & syrup. High sugar count.	230/8 oz
		KA

Photographs & Illustrations
Photo groups and montages are listed clockwise from top left corner of page.
Wikimedia Commons is online at http://commons.wikimedia.org/wiki/Main_Page

Chapter	Page	Name	Creator/Holder	Source
Cover		Aphrodite Anadyomene	Romeinse kopie naar een Grieks origineel Marmer, Musei Vaticani, Rome	Wikimedia Commons Public Domain from L.Sechan, art. Venus, in C Daremberg-E.Saglio, (edd)., Le Dictionnaire des Antiquites Grecques et Romaines, V, Parijs, 1904, p.724
Cover		Red Wine Glass	André Karwathaka	Wikimedia Creative Commons Attribution-Share Alike 2.5 Generic
Cover		Winter Wheat	Photographer: Michael Thompson	US Dept of Agriculture Public Domain Agricultural Research Service Photo Gallery Image No. K7394-6
Cover		Jug - Geometric oinoshoe Boetia, ca 750 BC	Photographer Jastrow, 2007 Louvre	Wikimedia Commons Public Domain
Cover		Bread loaf from "Bread Loaves"	Adam K. Thomas Seaman	Wikimedia Commons US Navy Public Domain
Cover		Grapes	PhotographerScott Bauer	US Dept of Agriculture Public Domain Photo Gallery Image No. K7248-1
1	1	Aphrodite Removing Her Sandal 1st century? Syria?	Louvre Museum Bronze with golden jewelry	Wikimedia Commons Public Domain
1	1	Birth of Venus Closeup 1482-1483	Sandro Botticelli	Wikimedia Commons Public Domain GNU Free Documentation License

1	1	Aphrodite Anadyomene (same as cover)	Romeinse kopie naar een Grieks origineel Marmer, Musei Vaticani, Rome	Wikimedia Commons Public Domain from L.Sechan, art. Venus, in C Daremberg-E.Saglio, (edd)., Le Dictionnaire des Antiquites Grecques et Romaines, V, Parijs, 1904, p.724
1	1	Aphrodite Kallipygos before 1914	Giorgio Sommer 1834-1914 Naples National Museum	Wikimedia Commons Public Domain
1	1	Madmoiselle Lange as Venus 1798	Anne-Louis Girodet de Roussy-Trioson	Wikimedia Commons Public Domain
1	1	Aphrodite Anadyomene from Pompeii Before 79CE Dug out in 1960	Ancient Rome artist. Photo by Steven Haynes. Possibly Roman copy of portrait of Campasne, mistress of Alexander the Great.	Wikimedia Commons Public Domain
1	2	Vulcan	Gillaume Cousteau the Younger, 1716-1777. Louvre Museum Marble Photographer Jastrow, 2006. Reception piece for French Royal Academy 1742. Seized during French Revolution	Wikimedia Commons Public Domain
1	2	Venus and Cupid (girdle belt)	Jan Saenredam , 1565-1607 & Hendrick Goltzius, 1558-1617 Engraving after Hendrick Goltzius	Wikimedia Commons Public Domain
1	2	Venus Aphrodite and Eros	Carlo Brogi 1850-1925 Rome National Museum	Wikimedia Commons Public Domain
1	3	Ares	Jastrow, 2006 Plaster replica of original stored at the	Wikimedia Commons Public Domain

			Museum of the Villa. Canope at the Villa Adriana in Tivoli.		
1	3	Adonis Led by Cupids to Venus 1600	Francesco Albani 1578-1660	Wikimedia Commons Public Domain
1	3	Adonis	19th century replica of a Greek bronze found at Pompeii. Museum of Naples. Photograph by fr. Utilisateur.DS	Wikimedia Commons GNU Free License Documentation
1	4	Death of Adonis	Giuseppe Mazzuoli ca. 1644-1725 Located at St. Petersburg Photograph Mark Thorpe, 1999	Wikimedia Commons Creative Attribution-Share Alike 2.5 Generic
1	4	Venus and Adonis 1637	Jose de Ribera Located at Deutsch: Galleria Nazionale di Palazzo Corsini	Wikimedia Commons Source: The Yorck Project, *10,000 Meisterwerke der Malerei*, DVD ROM, 2002. ISBN 3936122202, distributed by Directmedia Publishing GmBH. Compilation by Zenodof Verlagsgesellschat mbH GNU Free Documentation License
1	4	The Awakening of Adonis 1900	John William Waterhouse 1849-1917 Private Collection	Wikimedia Commons Public Domain Source: http://persephone.cps.unizar.es/General/Gente/SPD/Pre-Raphaelites/wat/jpg/water19.jpg
1	4	Statue of Isis-Persephone holding a sistrum	Wolfgang Sauber April 4, 2009 Archaeological Museum in Herakleion. Temple of the Eyptian	Wikimedia Commons GNU Free Documentation License, 1.2

			gods, Gortyn. Roman period (180-190 AC)	
1	5	Aphrodisias Tetrapylon	M.Chloe Mulderia Photo, Sept, 2004, taken in Turkey.	Wikimedia Commons Public domain.
1	6	Deutsch: Venus und Amor 1596	Johannes Rottenhammer 1564-1625	Wikimedia Commons Public Domain
1	6	Deutsch: Der Raub der Helena, Detail 1631	Guido Reni Louvre Museum	Wikimedia Commons Public Domain Source: The Yorck Project, *10,000 Meisterwerke der Malerei*, DVD ROM, 2002. ISBN 3936122202, distributed by Directmedia Publishing
1	6	Illustration to Ovid's Art of Love 1930	Jean de Bosschere The Love Books of Ovid	Wikimedia Commons Public Domain

Bibliography

Ancient Mesopotamian Foods. Ancient Egypt.
    http: www.foodtimeline.org/foodfaq3.html

Baines, Dr. John. *Ancient Egypt Timeline.*
    http: www.bbc.co.uk/history/ancient/egyptians/timeline.shtml

Billard, Jules B., Editor. *Ancient Egypt. Discovering its Splendors.* Washington, D.C.:
    National Geographic, 1978.

Hunter, Erica C.D. *First Civilizations*, Rev. Ed. New York: Facts on File, Inc. Oxfordshire,
    UK: Andromeda Oxford, Ltd., 2003.

Kirschmann, Gayla J., Nutrition Search, Inc., John D. Kirschmann, Director.
    Nutrition Almanac. 4th Edition. New York: McGraw-Hill, 1996.

Kirschmann, John D., Director, Nutrition Search, Inc. *Nutrition Almanac.* Rev. Ed.
    New York: McGraw-Hill, 1979.

Platt, Richard and Stephen Biesty. *Steven Biesty Cross-Sections Castle.* New York:
    Dorling Kindersley Publishing Inc., 1994.

U.S. Department of Agriculture. Agricultural Research Service. *Image Gallery &*
    Photo Library Archive. http://www.ars.usda.gov/is/graphics/photos/search.
    (2010)

U.S. Department of Agriculture. USDA Nutrient Data Laboratory.
    Food Composition. http: www.nal.usda.gov/fnic (Dec. 2003) (Jan.2010)

Wikimedia Commons (2010)
    http://commons.wikimedia.org/wiki/Main_Page

Wikipedia (2010)
    http://www.wikipedia.org/